THE ART AND SCIENCE OF CONNING DEPRESSION

MANIPULATING DEPRESSION AND EVERYTHING IT STANDS FOR

By

MODUPE LADELE

1st Edition 2022

Copyright © 2022

Photo by Ricardo Ortiz from Pexels

AOC

WHY YOU SHOULD READ THIS BOOK

Depression is eating through our world, it needs to be eradicated, we might be going through depression or maybe we have lost a loved one to it, probably through suicide or distancing by the depressed person.

Depression needs to be stopped, war needs to be waged against it, and we need to be able to snap out of that slippery slope called depression.

- The science around depression will be discussed

- The cause of depression will be discussed

- The manifestation of depression will be discussed

- How to con depression will be discussed

- Real-life and practical examples of how to con depression will be discussed

- How to win the war against depression will be discussed

- What you shouldn't do will be discussed

- Potential use of artificial intelligence and machine learning in eradicating depression will be discussed

- The reason for each discussion will be discussed

- Experiences and advice would be given.

Everything is a big con against depression, a journey, a major conspiracy against depression, and what it stands for, you are going to learn how to manipulate your depression.

Introduction

People who are not facing depression think that they understand what a depressed person is going through, apparently, because they have been down because they have been sad at one point in their lives they understand what being depressed is.

The google scholars, the talented google searchers who pose as self-made researchers, they go through the first three pages of Google or whatever search engine they are using, they open the first five search results, and read them and suddenly they think they understand what depression is.

It is not their fault, they are just trying to help in the best way they can, they can't understand unless they experience it and we not only hope to God but also pray to him that they don't experience it, I am not too bold to say "I wouldn't wish it on my worse enemy" I mean, they are called my worse enemy for a reason.

Please help me improve this book by contacting me
with suggestions and corrections, help this book
become better for someone else to read

TABLE OF CONTENTS

LEGAL NOTES

This book "The Art And Science Of Conning Depression" is not intended to be a substitution for professional advice, diagnosis, and/or treatment. Always seek the advice of your mental health professional or other qualified health providers with any questions you may have concerning your condition(s). You should never disregard professional advice(s)/instruction(s) or delay in seeking them because of something you read in this book.

You should note that only a licensed physician should evaluate your situation, provide a diagnosis, or render other medical advice to you.

What Is A Con?

A con according to the Oxford English dictionary is persuading (someone) to do or believe something by lying to them. It can be said to be an instance of deceiving or tricking someone, the people who do the activities are called con artists

"who is going to believe a con artist? Everyone, if she is good." – Andy Griffith

CAN DEPRESSION BE CONNED?

Short answer? Yes

Long answer? Well here we go

Depression is much more than an imbalance of chemicals in the brain. The cause of depression is a complex interplay of individual factors or multiple factors.

Apply that in conning depression will be that the prevention of depression would not be the appropriate point of entry during manipulation instead the effect would be the appropriate point of entry. In simpler terms, it is better to concentrate on solving the effects of depression than what causes it.

The reason is that a normal cause-and-effect relationship cannot be integrated into psychology concerning the exact cause of a patient's depression, that is because depression is caused by a lot of things, ranging from genetics to stress. Theoretically, deep learning a branch of machine learning can be somehow integrated into creating an algorithm for finding a pattern, to make a cause and effect relationship, but we will get to that.

This doesn't mean that one should not note and avoid the causes of depression if possible.

Since we are soon to be con artists, we should start from what we do know and that is the effects of depression, no matter the number of things that can cause depression, depression has similar effects. Meaning the cause would not be concentrated on and the con would be based on manipulating the effects.

If you are not convinced by this method, then you should know that the treatment of effect has an acceptable success rate even in modern medicine(sometimes while dealing with some sickness, the symptoms are being treated and not the sickness itself.) I noticed I was using one of the downfalls of modern medicine as a defence.

The idea of manipulation can be unsettling, but you should also know that manipulation is being used in different fields, I mean manipulation is one of the pillars of science if not the foundation (For example "when you reduce this, then what happens?" "What if you increase it, what happens?"). Osteopathic Manipulation Treatment(OMT) Doctors of osteopathy (Dos) literally take a hands-on approach to musculoskeletal disorders. Osteopathic manipulation treatment (OMT) is used to help correct structural imbalances in the body, improve circulation and relieve pain. There is manipulation in therapy, also in the treatment of spines, and so on.

WHAT IS DEPRESSION?

The first step in conning is studying your mark, I hope I did not write that statement because I watched "White Collar" that tv series is about a conman named Neal Caffrey, who is a criminal consultant for the white collar crime division of the FBI. I am starting to digress.

As I said, depression is killing our society slowly and because of that I once wrote a blog post about it on my previous blog, the title of that blog post was called "Depression And How To Help Eradicate It" I doubt you would find it because I mistakenly erased it from the internet, the whole blog and not just the post. Well, that was a blog post, this is a book.

You probably don't want to know what depression is because you know what exactly it is already, you more than know what it is, because you feel it.

Depression can be caused when neurotransmitters are little in the brain, these neurotransmitters help in relaying messages from each nerve cell in the brain, and it is believed that the messages they send play a role in mood regulation.

While applying a non-holistic and what one could refer to as an unconventional method of semi-reductionism in solving depression, this obviously goes against the famous notion that "What you don't know can't kill you" and closer to the "Repetition brings familiarity, and familiarity is the opposite of the unknown." By Steven Levenkron.

What better way to make the foundation than with a quote from Harry Potter and the Goblet of Fire "Understanding is the first step to acceptance, and only with acceptance can there be recovery."

If you read the book titled "How To Kill A Mockingbird" the phrase "Familiarity breeds contempt" will ring a bell, so let us get familiar with the science revolving around depression so it can lead to our contempt of depression on our part.

You might be currently experiencing depression or someone you care about is experiencing it so I am going to give what I can call a very detailed scientific and artistic explanation of what exactly depression is and the process it manifests itself, not that the science is the most important aspect but because it gives you a knowledge about it, and having that knowledge is key to opening the battle gate of where the war would be taken place between you "your majesty" and depression(I wonder what gender pronoun depression would like to be referred to).

Now that you know that understanding is the key to unlocking the battlefield for fighting depression you should also know that giving you the process that depression works help reduces it from the spirit that it is, to the ordinary chemical(s) that it manifests its self in.

Depression according to google is The persistent feeling of sadness or loss of interest. major depression can lead to a range of behavioral and physical symptoms. These may include changes in sleep, appetite, energy level, concentration, daily behaviour or self-esteem. Depression can also be associated with thoughts of suicide.

The purpose of this is to break down depression till its familiarity breeds contempt, I bet you are feeling more enlightened about your condition and I hope you are starting to contempt depression in all its forms.

Let us study the mark called depression a little bit more.

A mark is what a conman calls his target.

The Science Revolving Depression

According to Harvard Medical School through their platform 'Harvard health publishing' they said "It's often said that depression results from a chemical imbalance, but that figure of speech doesn't capture how complex the disease is. Research suggests that depression doesn't spring from simply having too much or too little of certain brain chemicals. Rather, there are many possible causes of depression, including faulty mood regulation by the brain, genetic vulnerability, and stressful life events. It's believed that several of these forces interact to bring on depression. To be sure, chemicals are involved in this process, but it is not a simple matter of one chemical being too low and another too high. Rather, many chemicals are involved, working both inside and outside nerve cells. There are millions, even billions, of chemical reactions that make up the dynamic system that is responsible for your mood, perceptions, and how you experience life."

Unlike love which is caused by a hormone called oxytocin or fear which is caused by a hormone called dopamine, depression is not caused by one or two chemicals, it is caused by many chemicals, hormones and a lot of other factors intrinsic or extrinsic to the host, host meaning the person going through depression, I like to think the chemicals are not responsible for depression but that the chemicals are one of the results of depression in the sense that it is how the brain reacts to such a complicated phenomenon, But what I like to think doesn't matter.

According to the endocrine web "*More research is needed around how hormones and mental health are connected, but experts say there is an interaction between hormones and well-being. Here's what we know: Your endocrine system works in tandem with your nervous system — known as the hypothalamic-pituitary system — to maintain a sense of homeostasis or physiological equilibrium. This equilibrium is what the body wants, but when it's not achieved, a lot can go wrong.*

When something is out of balance with your hormones it affects the whole system, which means you're going to feel it manifest both in your body and your mind.

Ready for a deeper dive? According to Dr Cory Rice, internist and certified BioTE practitioner, "The major endocrine glands in humans are the thyroid gland and the adrenal glands. If this chemical messaging system or the hormone feedback loops are negatively compromised in any way, this can have profound effects on someone's health, particularly as it relates to their mental health."

For example, he says, the thyroid gland is the "master gland" of our endocrine system. It's responsible for producing the hormones T3 and T4, and it's T3 that has a major role in one's mental health. "Many of the T3 receptors in our body are concentrated in our brain. So if we have a thyroid gland that is underperforming (not making enough T4 and/or T3), there is not enough thyroid hormone getting to the brain. This can, and oftentimes will lead to increased rates of depression or anxiety or other mental health issues."

For example, patients with hyperthyroidism and hypothyroidism can experience erratic and unpredictable mental states. Commonly reported are anxiety, brain fog, mania, lethargy, depressive mood, and confusion.

Dr Rice also explains that the adrenal glands help to regulate our internal stress response." If someone has physical, mental, or any other personal stress in their life, their adrenal glands may not function appropriately," he says. "Stress is very common for a lot of people. Some stress is good for us, but if certain types of stress persist for too long, this can have dramatic, detrimental effects on someone's health."

One of the hormones responsible for how we experience and manage stress? Cortisol. "If a person has consistent, uncontrolled stress, it will compromise their ability to produce and use their cortisol," Dr Rice says. "If this happens, they will oftentimes get very fatigued and gain weight — among other problems. This can also lead to mood disorders such as depression, apathy, and anxiety." "

When you suffer from depression, your brain is physically changed. Research by the National Institutes of Health shows that you lose grey matter volume (GMV) when you suffer from depression. This loss is caused by parts of your brain shrinking due to the hormone cortisol impeding the growth of your brain cells. The more serious depression a person suffers, the more GMV they lose. Since GMV contains most of your neurons or nerve cells, slowed growth means that your cognitive capabilities are at risk of impairment. The hippocampus raises its cortisol levels, impeding the development of neurons in your brain, other cerebral areas shrink due to high levels of cortisol, and the amygdala enlarges. The amygdala controls emotion, so this may cause issues like sleep disturbances, mood swings, and other hormone-related problems. An enlarged amygdala is also linked to the development of the bipolar disorder.

Major depression is linked to cerebral inflammation. While there's no solid evidence from experts on whether depression causes cerebral inflammation or vice versa, A Causality paradox at its very core, taking stress as an example; stress can cause high blood pressure which is a condition in which the force of blood against the artery walls is too high, which can lead to heart attacks or strokes which generally causes a shortage of oxygen to the brain and since a chronic lack of oxygen can cause inflammation in the body's tissue, it is only logical that it does the same to the brain, which supports what I initially said, "**I like to think the chemicals are not responsible for depression but that the chemicals are one of the results of depression in the sense that it is how the brain reacts to such a complicated phenomenon, But what I like to think doesn't matter.**"

Whatever the extrinsic cause is, it manifests itself as an intrinsic cause, I guess that what I like to think does matter, and maybe it is not that much of a causality paradox.

Better researchers have posited that these two are closely linked. Studies found that people who have suffered depression for over ten years experience 30% more cerebral inflammation compared to those who suffer from a shorter period of depression. Since cerebral inflammation kills neurons, it can lead to many complications. The death of neurons and neurotransmitters may lead to shrinkage as well as reduce a person's neuroplasticity – the ability of brains to change as the person ages. Since new neurons and neurotransmitters will have a tougher time growing, this leads to cognitive problems in the affected person.

We can't help but wonder what the source of depression is and what the potential causes may be.

Everything can be simplified to the problem in the communication within the neurons of your brain, the secret can be the enhanced glutamate production, it can be a balance in the dopamine hormone and if you are into tech, it can be a collection of data on how different receptors in the brain of various non-depressed hosts using brain mapping devices, cleaning of the collected data, using it to train a machine learning model till an acceptable percentage of probability is derived and somehow implement it into correcting the receptors in the brain of depressed hosts there will be a need to take care of some new logic along the way but one must be careful so as not to play God because the consequence is destruction.

TYPES OF DEPRESSION

1) Major depressive disorder: It is commonly known and referred to as clinical depression, unipolar depression or simply 'depression' and it is characterized by the following.

i) Anhedonia: Lack of interest in activities normally enjoyed.

ii) Changes in weight: loss or gain in weight

iii) Changes in sleep: irregular sleeping

iv) Fatigue

v) Feelings of worthlessness, despair and guilt

vi) Difficulty concentrating

vii) Thoughts of death and suicide

viii) Depress mood/ Low mood

2) Persistent depressive disorder: It is mild and long-lasting you can have it and not know. According to

 Persistent depressive disorder, also called dysthymia (dis-THIE-me-uh), is a continuous long-term (chronic) form of depression. You may lose interest in normal daily activities, feel hopeless, lack productivity, and have low self-esteem and an overall feeling of inadequacy. These feelings last for years and may significantly interfere with your relationships, school, work and daily activities.

If you have a persistent depressive disorder, you may find it hard to be upbeat even on happy occasions — you may be described as having a gloomy personality, constantly complaining or incapable of having fun. Though the persistent depressive disorder is not as severe as major depression, your current depressed mood may be mild, moderate or severe.

It's your birthday but you don't know what the fuss is all about, it can be adulthood, it can be a persistent depressive disorder, it can be both and who knows maybe adulthood is persistent depressive disorder (JJ).

3) Bipolar Disorder: it can also be referred to as a manic depression. A disorder associated with episodes of mood swings ranging from depressive lows to manic highs.

The exact cause of the bipolar disorder isn't known, but a combination of genetics, environment and altered brain structure and chemistry may play a role. Manic episodes may include symptoms such as high energy, reduced need for sleep and loss of touch with reality. Depressive episodes may include symptoms such as:

- Low energy
- Low motivation
- Loss of interest in daily activities.

Mood episodes last days to months at a time and may also be associated with suicidal thoughts.

4) Seasonal Affective Disorder: SAD the acronym and the feeling, it is a disorder that helps value the sun, the affected party shines when the sun shines.

A mood disorder characterized by depression that occurs at the same time every year.

The seasonal affective disorder occurs in climates where there is less sunlight at certain times of the year.

Symptoms include:

Fatigue, depression, hopelessness and social withdrawal.

Mood: anxiety, apathy, general discontent, loneliness, loss of interest, mood swings, or sadness

Sleep: excess sleepiness, insomnia, or sleep deprivation

Whole body: appetite changes or fatigue

Behavioural: irritability or social isolation

Also common: Depression, lack of concentration, or weight gain.

It is a type of depression so google did not have to tell us depression is also a symptom of SAD.

5) Psychotic Depression: Also known as depressive psychosis, is a major depressive episode that is accompanied by psychotic symptoms (Hales and

Yudofsky, 2003). It can occur in the context of bipolar disorder or major depressive disorder. (Hales and Yudofsky, 2003) It can be difficult to distinguish from schizoaffective disorder, a diagnosis that requires the presence of psychotic symptoms for at least two weeks without any mood symptoms present. (Hales and Yudofsky, 2003) Unipolar psychotic depression requires that the psychotic features occur only during episodes of major depression. Diagnosis using the DSM-5 involves meeting the criteria for a major depressive episode, along with the criteria for a "mood-congruent or mood-incongruent psychotic features" specifier. (American Psychiatric Association, 2013)

6) Postpartum depression: Depression that occurs after childbirth.
Those who develop postpartum depression are at greater risk of developing major depression later on in life.

Symptoms:

- Insomnia, loss of appetite, intense irritability and difficulty bonding with the baby.
- Mood: anger, anxiety, guilt, hopelessness, loss of interest or pleasure in activities, mood swings, or panic attack.
- Behavioural: crying, irritability, or restlessness.
- Whole body: fatigue or loss of appetite.
- Weight: weight gain or weight loss.
- Cognitive: lack of concentration or unwanted thoughts.
- Psychological: depression or fear.
- Also common: is insomnia or rumination.

There are many types of depression, many are not listed here, but the truth is that the method of war for one applies to all, what I mean is that the same way to wage and win the war against SAD is the same way you wage and win the war against MDD and the rest.

Signs Of Depression

A depressed person will probably not know they are depressed.

Deep feelings of sadness: This happens in the sense that an overwhelming sadness with or without cause happens, just that deep dark well.

Dark moods: Some very dark moods appear like a reaction to things and how one behaves.

Feelings of worthlessness or hopelessness: Felling of not being important enough that nothing good can ever happen again.

Appetite changes: Noticed that I didn't say the loss of appetite, I said appetite changes because it can happen in the form of having a loss of appetite or one can start binge eating.

Sleep changes: Sleeping schedules become disoriented

Lack of energy: Lost of energy to perform the basic act, eat something with high calories and for some reason, you don't have strength.

Inability to concentrate: You are often in your head, so you are unable to concentrate on anything.

Difficulty getting through your normal activities: It becomes harder to get through your normal activities

Others: Lack of interest in things you used to enjoy The things you use to enjoy seem boring, withdrawing from friends(you want to be alone so you withdraw from your circle), thinking a lot about death or self-harm(You think about doing yourself harm or killing yourself).

Cause Of Depression

We know that depression is a complex disease, the cause can be from genetics to illness.

The various causes of depression can be;

- Stressful events
- Family history
- Giving birth
- Loneliness
- Alcohol and drugs
- Illness
- Poor nutrition.
- Unresolved grief or loss.
- Personality traits.
- Medication and substance use
- Noise pollution

These are some of the known causes of depression, what all these causes have in common is their effect. Let us talk about them.

Stressful events: Sometimes we do somethings that get us stressed, maybe it is out 7-5 jobs, maybe it is caring for some of our loved one in need or whatever it may be, when we get stressed the body responds to it, your heart rate increases, breathing quickens, muscles tighten, and blood pressure rises, when the heart rate increases what happens? It may not pump enough blood to the rest of the body. As a result, the organs and tissues may not get enough oxygen. In general, tachycardia. An increase in heart rate means an increase in heartbeat and if the brain is part of the organs not getting enough oxygen, then inflammation starts to occur in the brain.
Encephalitis is inflammation of the active tissues of the brain caused by an infection or an autoimmune response(the autoimmune response in this case is an automatic response to stressful events). The inflammation causes the brain to swell, which can

lead to headaches, stiff neck, sensitivity to light, mental confusion and seizures. It is also possible that a drop in the brain pressure occurs and that can cause a constant throbbing headache which may be worse in the morning, or when coughing or straining, it also causes sick-like effects of not wanting to go out, loss of appetite and so on. All this is enough to cause a major disequilibrium in the brain hormones which is one of the things we first learnt about depression (" depression results from a chemical imbalance")

Family History: A lot of things can be passed down from a parent to offspring, to learn more about the research you can just read about Mendel and his research. To do a little justice to this book, we should know that heart disease, high blood pressure, Alzheimer's disease, arthritis, diabetes, cancer, and obesity can be passed through generations, those seven listed are even called the "Seven common multifactorial genetic inheritance disorders" those diseases are can be associated with depression so it

makes sense that depression to can be passed down
from one generation to another.

In psychology, genetic memory is a theorized
phenomenon in which certain kinds of memories
could be inherited, being present at birth. I did not say
that, Wikipedia did. Someone said phobia is what
caused the death of an offspring's ancestor. I am not
sure, but someone somewhere might have said it.

My point is this If things like that can be passed from
a parent to an offspring then many other things can
be passed on within a family.

Let's take an unexpected angle at Family history, it
has been said that "People whose handwriting is
extremely similar to their parents didn't inherit it they
simply copied it, maybe even subconsciously." this
means that sometimes when children have depressed
and it can be traced to the parents or a family
member they are often with there is a possibility that it
caused by a subconscious imitation, this can also
explain why peer group behaviour or the world at
large can cause depression.

Giving birth: Lochia, is also called vaginal discharge, it is bleeding from the vagina and it occurs to the mother after the first few days of childbirth, like I said earlier your body responds to things, Lochia is the body of a woman that just gave birth getting rid of the blood and tissue that was inside her uterus. For the first few days, the blood is heavy and bright red, after some time, the flow gets less and the blood colour is lighter, if for some reason the amount of blood loss is more than it should be then the blood pressure falls it can lead to people being dizzy, people may be tired, short of breath may occur, and there can be paleness. When the loss of blood is a little more than that then the low blood pressure can reduce the body's oxygen levels, which can lead to enough oxygen not reaching the brain. more than that again can lead to dizziness and fainting. let us focus on the "lead to enough oxygen not reaching the brain" we both know what that can cause. Note Lochia will not cause oxygen to not reach the brain but may cause oxygen to not reach the brain. The chances are small, the odds are little, but when you place those odds on the current population of the world then you begin to understand why it happens to some people.

Loneliness: We talked about the causality paradox, and this may seem like one because "has one's mental health made him/her lonely or has loneliness damaged his/her mental health" I think it is not too tricky to be labelled a causality paradox and if I think it is not tricky, then I already have the answer, which I am planning to share with you later on in this book. Research suggests that loneliness is associated with an increased risk of certain mental health problems, including depression, anxiety, low self-esteem, sleep problems and increased stress.

If you are lonely, you eat more which can lead to high cholesterol and/or diabetes based on the type of food you decided to eat more. High cholesterol is when you have too much of a fatty substance called cholesterol in your blood. It's mainly caused by eating fatty food, not exercising enough, being overweight, smoking and drinking alcohol which is what can happen when loneliness occurs. This can lead to a heart condition, and we all know what it might also lead to which will somehow lead to inflammation of the brain and/or imbalance of hormones in the brain.

Alcohol and drugs: Alcohol can lead to high cholesterol, if you are sceptical about alcohol leading to cholesterol I understand. I have friends who talk about how alcohol helps to burn down body fat and can even be used in weight reduction programs. I can neither confirm nor deny what some of my friends say about alcohol and its effect on body fat (I am starting to think I would make a good lawyer) but being fat and having high cholesterol are two different things. When you drink alcohol, while it may or may not be burning the body fat, alcohol is broken down and rebuilt into triglycerides and cholesterol in the liver. So, drinking alcohol raises the triglycerides and cholesterol in your blood. If your triglyceride levels become too high, they can build up in the liver, causing fatty liver disease. It can also lead to an increase in blood pressure which we both know how it may somehow lead to depression.

Drugs, on the other hand, can be very dangerous especially when not prescribed by a medical professional, even ketamine when used alone can cause a lot of things.

When higher doses of ketamine are abused, or during emergence, it is reported to produce vivid dreams and an "out-of-body", "K-hole" or "near-death" hallucinogenic experience, often reported as terrifying (similar to a bad LSD trip). If you know what a bad LSD trip is then you would understand how bad ketamine can be when abused.

When ketamine is used in smaller doses it can cause;

- Feelings of calmness and relaxation

- Relief from pain

- Depressed mental state

- Dizziness

- Detached feeling from the body

- Slurred speech

- Diminished reflexes

- Hallucinations lasting from 30 to 60 minutes

- Nystagmus (repetitive, uncontrolled movements of the eyes).

Abuse of ketamine can be linked with short-term and long-term problems:

Short-term;
- Problems with attention, learning, and memory
- Dreamlike states
- Hallucinations
- Sedation
- Confusion
- Loss of memory
- Raised blood pressure
- Unconsciousness
- Dangerously slowed breathing.

Long-term;
- Ulcers and pain in the bladder
- Kidney problems
- Stomach pain

- Depression

- Poor memory.

The reason I am talking about Ketamine specifically is that on March 5, 2019, the Food and Drug Administration (FDA) approved the first new medication for major depression in decades. The drug is a nasal spray called esketamine, derived from ketamine—an anaesthetic that has made waves for its surprising antidepressant effect.
If ketamine of all drugs can cause this, then taking drugs exposes people to a lot of things, it can lead to addiction, lead to depression, lead to insanity, and it can also lead to death.

Illness: The way the body reacts to illness can lead to depression, the symptoms of this illness can also be things that lead to depression.
An estimated one-third of people with serious chronic illness experience symptoms of depression, it has also been said by researchers that chronic illness can sometimes be a trigger to depression.

Poor nutrition: Not eating healthy food is bad, eating a lot of fatty food can lead to high cholesterol which can lead to depression, not eating good food can sometimes lead to stress which can lead to depression.

When some nutrients are missing in the body and we eat food that is also lacking these nutrients it can cause a subconscious increase in food intake to somehow complement this missing nutrient, the increase in food intake can lead to things that can lead to depression. Also when we are unable to get said nutrient the body might not act as it should, which can cause the body to not react like it should which we both know is bad and might lead to depression

Unresolved grief or loss: Not all unresolved griefs lead to depression, but still some do, the reason is that based on personality type, environment, upbringing and other things that make one human distinct from the other, we as humans react differently to unresolved grief or loss, one can decide to drown the grief or loss in alcohol to later find that grief and better swimmers than whoever won the best swimmer in the Guinness book of record. They can decide to engage in drugs, which can lead to depression, they can decide to swamp themselves with work to distract them which can lead to stress, then might somehow lead to depression and so on

Personality traits: Relations entre traits de personnalité et dépression au niveau des cinq grands facteurs et de leurs facettes, a research paper writen by Rajaa Jourdy, Jean-Michel Petot in 2017, the what they found out was this; Their findings confirmed the personality profile for depression suggested by Kotov et al. (2010) in their meta-analysis. Moreover, for the facets, they found significant differences between depressed participants and the French validation sample on at least one facet of every Big Five factor. These findings are largely comparable to the literature in that area, although differences in the facets of

Openness and Agreeableness were not exactly those that were expected. The correlation analyses additionally suggested that, for the Big Five domains as well as for the facets, there is a continuous linear association between severity of depression and Neuroticism and Conscientiousness, but not Extraversion, Openness, or Agreeableness. These associations are mainly related to four facets of Neuroticism (Angry Hostility, Depression, Self-Consciousness, and Vulnerability) and two facets of Conscientiousness (Competence and Self-Discipline). As this study was cross-sectional, it does not enable conclusions as to whether this profile was present before the onset of the depressive episode or appeared afterwards. However, it is suggested, based on the literature, that this profile could be premorbid and thereafter accentuated by acute depression. Their conclusion;

"Whatever the answer to this question, we can assume that a current depressive episode is strongly associated with a specific personality profile, including not only Neuroticism, Extraversion, and

Conscientiousness, but also two facets of Openness to Experience (Openness to Actions and Openness to Values) and one facet of Agreeableness (Trust)."
In simpler terms, there is a relationship between depression and personality traits.

Medication and substance use: We already know what taking unprescribed drugs can cause. Also, prescribed drugs can have side effects, a lot of drugs have a lot of possible side effects, and some of these side effects can have the same symptoms as depression or can cause depression.
Since some drugs are antidepressants it only makes sense that some can be prodepressants or at least their side effects can be.

Noise pollution: People underestimate the power of noise, research has proven that noise pollution can cause depression, it might even explain why people who are shouted upon as children might have depression.

The influence of noise on human cognitive performance and brain activity has been often neglected (Basner et al., 2014). Noise has different negative effects ranging from interference with cognitive processing to damaging mental and physical health (Stansfeld & Matheson., 2003). The World Health Organization (WHO) estimates that at least 1 million healthy life-years (disability-adjusted life-years) are lost annually as a result of environmental noise in high-income western European nations (with a population of around 340 million) (Basner., et al 2014). Studies show that noise causes cognitive impairment and oxidative stress in the brain (Wang et al., 2016). According to Wang et al., 2016 with further urbanization and industrialization, noise pollution has become a risk factor for depression, cognitive impairment and neurodegenerative disorders (Wang et al., 2016).

When there is the noise the body reacts by releasing cortisol which is a stress hormone, which can cause disbalance or hormone or can denote stress which we both know might lead to depression.

THE BATTLE WITH DEPRESSION

The reason there is a page title called the battle with depression is that, this book had a lot of titles, How To Fight Against Depression, How To Con Depression, Conning Your Way Out of Depression, Imprisoning Depression before I later went along with "The Art And Science Of Conning Depression"

Depression is a bitchy little thing that affects the body and mind, it makes you unwilling to fight, it is an ever sinking well with drowning being its evitable end."Note: EVITABLE END"
The secret is when you start to fight it, the battle is half won.
Depression in the sense that I hate that it is slowly eating our world today, it is affecting great and small, rich and poor, the famous ones are not immune to it, it doesn't just bring a strain on the affected individual it also affects the individual's friend and family.

There are a lot of things that can be added to this book, there are things that can be removed from this book, help make this book by reaching out to me to inform me of what you think might help this book better.

"Ona Kan o wo oja" a Yoruba saying that literally translates to one way doesn't lead to the market, you would understand this better if you have ever been to a Nigerian market, in the sense that there are various ways to enter a market, well there are several things that bring on depression and luckily for you, there are various ways to con depression.

CONNING DEPRESSION

CON ONE

Like I said earlier, waging war against depression
means you are halfway winning the battle and how
can you wage war against depression.

**Stand up and say to yourself depression is no
more**

Yup, I know it is a cheesy thing to say, but it does
work after you say that while standing up of course
one of two things happen:
You know deep down that depression isn't here to
stay, the unwillingness to fight is starting to fade
away.

OR

You find it too cheesy but you can help but blush, while you repeat it over and over, you are making a joke of depression, its reign is almost over in you. So don't be shy at depression, say to it over and over "depression no more"
Now the fact that your limps don't work doesn't mean you cannot stand up to depression all you need to do is to imagine yourself standing up and speck those words you can even imagine yourself sitting on depression and start telling it "DEPRESSION NO MORE"

The science: Studies prove that positive affirmations help activate parts of the brain that are associated with self-related processing and reward.
Under the Oxford University Press concerning the Social Cognitive and Affective Neuroscience an article by Christopher N.Cascio and others proved that Self-affirmation activates brain systems associated with self-related processing and reward and is reinforced by future orientation. These guys are good at what

they do so I am hoping you would just take their word

for it.

<u>CON TWO</u>

Challenge negative thoughts

You already told depression "NO More" and that is challenging depression itself, another important thing to do is to challenge the fruit of depression which is negative thoughts.
Understanding how your mind works can be key to challenging negative thoughts in the sense that when you understand your thought pattern you would be able to redirect it to positive thoughts.
Also, you can try out the things that can cause positive thoughts like being grateful for everything, it might be tough to be grateful for everything so check out this example
A man in a car with air conditioning sees a man in a car with no air conditioning and goes thank you lord that I have a car with air conditioning, the other man with no air conditioning sees someone riding a bicycle

to the work and goes, thank God I have a car, the man riding a bicycle sees someone walking to work and goes 'thank God I have a bike' the man on the bike saw a man walking and goes 'thank God I have a bike' the man walking saw a man on the wheelchair and goes 'thank God I have legs' the man on the wheelchair saw a dead man and goes 'thank God I am alive'
If you are reading this, you are not dead and I am certain about that because like google has it are you a robot checkbox, I also have my are you alive checkbox, it can only be seen by the dead(I hope you know I'm joking)(Well unless I am not)

There is always something to be thankful for.

Another way in challenging negative thoughts is to imagine yourself literally removing or redirecting negative energy and then absorbing positive energy. You can challenge negative thoughts by laughing at silly things you do when you are alone, and surround yourself with positive people because that positivity

has a way of rubbing off on you and helping others,
this explains why meditation works.

<u>CON THREE</u>

Exercise

Scientifically when you exercise depression would be eased and reduced by easing depression and anxiety by Releasing feel-good endorphins, natural cannabis-like brain chemicals (endogenous cannabinoids) and other natural brain chemicals that can enhance your sense of well-being.

After being chased by a dog or mother hen every feeling would leave you for the next 30 minutes give or take, you should trust that fact, it is from my personal experience.

There is evidence to suggest that the addition of cognitive-behavioural therapies, specifically exercise, can improve treatment outcomes for many depressed people. Exercise is a behavioural intervention that has shown great promise in alleviating symptoms of depression.

Involvement in structured exercise has shown promise in alleviating symptoms of clinical depression. Since the early 1900s, researchers have been interested in the association between exercise and depression. Early case studies concluded that, at least for some, moderate-intensity exercise should be beneficial for depression and result in a happier mood.15,16 Further, a relationship between physical work capacity (PWC) and depression appeared to exist,11–1 but the directional nature of this relationship could not be addressed via a case and cross-sectional studies. However, researchers have remained interested in the antidepressant effects of exercise and more recently have utilized experimental designs to study this association.

You might not want to believe in all scientific things but try it out consistently for three days and when it works don't forget to continue.

Examples of exercises to try out are:

1) Go for a run for an all-natural mood boost
2) Jogging: away depression
3) Walking: away from depression
4) Lift some weight: to lift your mood

5) Practice yoga: to (think of something creative to use here I am out of ideas :))

Jokes

You don't need a scientific reason for while jokes can help, jokes are fun, let us try some.

1. There's a fine line between a numerator and a denominator. (...Only a fraction of people will get this clean joke.)

2. What do dentists call their x-rays?

Tooth pics!

3. Did you hear about the first restaurant to open on the moon?

It had great food, but no atmosphere.

4. What did one <u>ocean</u> say to the other ocean?

Nothing, it just waved.

5. Do you want to hear a construction joke?

Sorry, I'm still working on it.

6. Did you hear about the fire at the circus?
It was in tents!

7. Why do ducks have feathers?

To cover their butt quacks!

8. What's the difference between a hippo and a zippo?

One is heavy and the other's a little lighter.

9. What does a nosey pepper do?

It gets jalapeño business.

10. Why should you never trust stairs?

They're always up to something.

Since I can't just copy and paste all the jokes on the internet here, I will paste links on where to find them. I gave you ten fish and I'm still about to teach you how to catch more fish, I am a hell of a fisherman/fisherman coach.

https://www.womansday.com/life/entertainment/a38635408/corny-jokes/

https://www.rd.com/list/funniest-jokes-of-all-time/

https://parade.com/1041830/marynliles/clean-jokes/

https://www.readersdigest.ca/culture/funny-jokes-national-tell-joke-day/

Don't settle on jokes alone, you can read joke stories, they are funny short jokes that will make you laugh, let the fisherman fish you some examples:

1) Akpos called his girlfriend, Joy, on phone, but unfortunately her father, an Army General picked up the call:

General: Hello! May I know you?

Caller (Akpos): Sorry I want to speak with Joy, sir.

General: I said who are you and why are you calling my daughter?

Akpos: (Akpos knew he had to act fast) Okay Sir, I am FRANK EDOHO from WHO WANTS TO BE A MILLIONAIRE. Joy's friend is presently on the hot seat and needs her help to answer a question for 2 Million Naira. So

the next voice you hear after is hers, the time starts now.......

General: Ooh am very sorry!!! Joy! Joy!! Pls take your phone your friend needs your help..........

Akpos: The question is, when are you coming to tomorrow? A. Morning, B. Afternoon, C.Evening, D. Night. Joy: D. Night.

Akpos: Are you sure? Final answer?.

Joy: Yes am very sure!

Akpos: okay, greet that father of yours for me.

2) In an external examination, the invigilator saw that Akpos had written some mathematical formula on his hands. The following conversation ensued:

Invigilator: Why did you write the formulas on your hand?

AKPOS: My teacher told us that formulas must be at your fingertips.

3) Young man, you are coming to seek my daughter's hand in marriage and you are chewing gum.

That's a sign of disrespect!

Akpos: Sir, I only chew gum when I drink or smoke.

Father-In-Law: You mean you drink and smoke and you are here to seek my daughter's hand in marriage?

Akpos: Sir I only drink and smoke when I go to the club.

Father-In-Law: You club too?

Akpos: I'm sorry sir, I started clubbing when I came out of prison.

Father-In-Law: You've also been in prison before? Oh my God!

Akpos: Sorry sir, I went to jail when I killed somebody!!

Father-In-Law: What!!! You're a killer and you want me to give you my daughter's hand in marriage?

Akpos: Sir, it happened out of anger. It was a certain man that didn't allow me to marry his daughter, so I killed him.
Father-In-Law: You are highly welcome my son. You are on the right track. You are absolutely the right man for my daughter.

4) The following conversation ensued between Akpos and Emeka.
Emeka: Why do you hold your wife's hand when you visit shopping malls?
Akpos: Because if I leave her hand she'll go shopping. It looks "ROMANTIC" but actually, it's "ECONOMIC".

5) Akpos went to Church on Sunday and gave testimony that he was infected with Ebola and that God had healed him.
When he finished, he tried to give the microphone to the second man who was waiting to give his testimony, but the man refused to take it:

The following conversation ensued:

2nd man – I have no testimony. Give it to Pastor.

(Akpos tried to give the microphone to the Pastor)

Pastor – I'm not in charge of testimonies so give it to the Senior Pastor.

(Akpos goes to the Senior Pastor)

Senior Pastor – Brother in Christ, the mic is yours. It's a gift from the Church. You may take it home.

And how to fish for them

https://thoughtcatalog.com/january-nelson/2018/06/funny-stories/

https://thefunnybeaver.com/15-really-funny-short-stories/

https://blog.reedsy.com/short-stories/funny/

you can also search "Akpos Jokes" on any search engine you use.

Now the trick is not in reading the jokes or funny storytelling them to another person is nice.

<u>CON FIVE</u>

Music

"Life is one grand, sweet song, so start the music."
Ronald Reagan definitely knew what he was talking
about because according to John Paul Friedrich
Richter "Music is the moonlight in the gloomy night of
life."
We all know the power that is in music, we know of its
ability to heal the spirit and uplift the mood. I am not
telling you to go listen to some dark or sad song I am
telling you to listen to a song that will inspire you,
uplift you and any other song that is fun and you can
dance to.
If you like science then check this out:
A Harvard research study that dissected the
relationship between music and mental health notes
that an authoritative review of research performed
between 1994 and 1999 reported that in four trials,
music therapy reduced symptoms of depression,

while a fifth study found no benefit. It worked four times out of five, that is a good outcome.

Listening to the wrong choice of music is worse than not listening to music at all as it can increase depression so I am going to give you a list of songs you should listen to

1) Hello by Martin Solveig & Dragonette
2) As many songs as possible by NF (you can start with the album titled therapy)
3) C major by Seyi Vibez
4) Song of Angels by Judikay
5) Kaabo (welcome) by Dunsin Oyekan
6) Ainsi bas la vida(bonus track) by Indila
7) Yeshua Hamashiach by Nathaniel Bassey
8) Rock your body by Burna boy
9) Anybody by Burna boy
10) On the low by Burna boy
11) Winterbird by Lùisa
12) Parle À Ta Tête by Indila
13) Reckless Love by Cory Asbury

Check out all these songs, especially song number 13, I had to save the best for the last. And if you need any other recommendations just contact me.

I find Hello by Martin Solveig & Dragonette to be a great song, to me, it is a song about a young woman who is at a party to have fun, she is not there to start something, she is probably involved with someone, she flirts with this guy who she finds kind of cute, but she is just having her fun, nothing more, the guy is expecting more, he is alright but she just came to enjoy the party.

NF is something else, that is all I can say, but try to listen to his songs, you would love them.

C major by Seyi Vibez is a Nigerian song that talks about Things like God, money, and life and are filled with vibes. 98% vibes.

Song of Angels by Judikay is a must listen, it takes you to that heavenly ream that you have to experience before you can understand, it is truly the song of angels, it references the all mighty God, the creator.

Kaabo (welcome) by Dunsin Oyekan is a song that talks about the presence of God in a gathering, how to welcome God the king of glory, you don't have to heaven to experience God, you can bring him here.

Ainsi bas la vida(bonus track) by Indila is a french song about love with a broken stranger, listen to it and you will think it is much more than that, who knows maybe it is.

Yeshua Hamashiach by Nathaniel Bassey is talking about the lion of Judah, trust me you would want to know about him.

Rock your body by Burna boy is a vibe, it talks about this girl that thinks she is bad, she said her man can't control her body and that her body should be rocked. I think she has misguided feminism syndrome.

Anybody by Burna boy, the energy in this song is something else

On the low by Burna boy, what I am going to say about this song is that depression gots nothing against this song.

Winterbird by Lùisa, I fell in love with Lùisa at a particular scene in orange is the new black, when a prison break just happened, and the water was splashing and her song was playing " Under The Wild Skies" I had to look up who that musician was.
Well, Winterbird by Lùisa talks about her search for someone or something or who knows maybe herself.

Parle À Ta Tête by Indila in my opinion is talking about; talking yourself out of depression

Reckless Love by Cory Asbury, like I said I saved the best for the last, imagine the creator(The one who made us and where we live) imagine that creator loving you so much that he is willing to do what you don't deserve, willing to do (Imagine them) well talk about imaginations come true.

The science: When music is played, the vibration travels through the brain and tickles the eardrum and is transmitted into an electric signal that travels through the auditory nerve to the brain stem, where is reassembled into something we perceive as music. Sugaya and Yonetani. Recent studies found out that playing someone's favourite music, different parts of the brain light up.

<u>CON SIX</u>

Watch a comedy series

Comedy series is fun, there are helpful with depression, now make sure you watch them in moderation, no excessive watching of comedy series. The reason I made mention of series and not movies is that comedy series work better than comedy movies, examples of comedy series that I can recommend to you are the following

1) How I met your mother
2) The office
3) Ted lasso (especially if you are a football fan) (I believe you Americans call it soccer)
4) The big bang theory (imagine not having a friend like Sheldon is enough to lift you from depression, if you think I am lying just watch the show)
5) Seinfeld (this is legendary)

As usual, the best for the last so number five. Remember no excessive watching. Watch them yourself I am not planning to explain them to you, all I can say is to reach out to me when you are watching, watch with a loved one.

<u>CON SEVEN</u>

Eat healthily

Seems like I have hit a nerve with all the junks you have been taking recently. Well, healthy eating is key to having a depression-free life. The brain needs some nutrients to function well, and you can't get those nutrients from junk

Now the science of it;

A 2017 study by Trusted Source found that the symptoms of people with moderate-to-severe depression improved when they received nutritional counselling sessions and ate a more healthful diet for 12 weeks. The improved diet focused on fresh and whole foods that are high in nutrients. It also limited processed refined foods, sweets, and fried food, including junk food. The researchers concluded that people could help manage or improve their symptoms of depression by addressing their diet. (Jon Johnson on August 20, 2019)

Had fruit to your diet, simply go monk mode, and do experiments with different vegetables, the experiment is making new food can be fun in itself.

<u>CON EIGHT</u>

Set attainable and realistic goals

I did not say to you set goals, I said set attainable and
realistic goals, not just any goals but attainable and
realistic ones.
It can also serve as a distraction to help you reach
achieving that goal, also it can be fulfilling when you
reach those goals.
When you set goals, it gives one a sense of purpose
and the truth is when there is a purpose, there is a
rebirth in an existing life, so set some goals and make
sure they are realistic goals and also attainable.
Your brain rewards you when you achieve your goals.

<u>CON NINE</u>

Reward your effort

When you reach those attainable and realistic goals
that I mentioned earlier you need to reward your
effort, it is a way of finding joy in the little things.
Take yourself out on a date, no human can take care
of you better than yourself.
Get yourself a gift and wrap it up, there is this funny
video of Mr Bean that I watched a long time ago, he
wrapped up a gift, then placed it outside his door
entered his house back and pretended he heard a
knock, he then opened the door, looked around saw
the gift, picked it up, came back to his house
unwrapped it and acted surprised throughout the
process. No wonder he is happy he knows have to
get something for himself and also put up a show
while doing it.

<u>CON TEN</u>

Spend time with your love once

They love you and they want the best for you, so spend time with them, entertain them, have fun with them, and do something you enjoy doing together.

You know some of that jokes and the funny story you read, tell it to them, listen to some of that music with them, watch some of those series with them, talk about it with them.

Many people have someone that when they talk to, they feel happy

But what you must do is that with all your might resist that feeling to segregate yourself from those that love you, fight that spirit of loneliness.

<u>CON ELEVEN</u>

Help someone out/Make someone happy

You can distract yourself by helping someone out with something, helping them can or making them happy, helping someone or/and making someone happy makes us happy too, this is because the creator has wired us in a way that helping people out makes us happy.
"The purpose of human life is to serve and to show compassion and the will to help others," Albert Schweitzer.
The science of it right? The same hormone that is secreted while exercising is also secreted when you help people out or make someone else happy, the hormone is called Endorphins.
Go out of your way to help someone in need, give out something to someone in need, you helping them out helps you a great deal.

You would not be only doing good to the world, you would also be destroying the bitchy little thing called depression.

<u>CON TWELVE</u>

Get enough sleep

Sleep is very important, I know that oversleeping can cause depression and worsen depression somethings but it doesn't cause depression. Some studies show that people with insomnia have a higher risk of having depression. Get enough sleep, not excess sleep and not little sleep enough sleep, 8 hours of sleep.

<u>CON THIRTEEN</u>

Visit your therapist

The disclaimer in this book is enough to tell you why
you should visit your therapist. They studied for years
to help people.
What a cool job to have, helping people and making
money in the process.

BEST FOR THE LAST

Meet with the master healer

Well, you know me, always saving the best for the last.
People often underestimate not only the power but the love that the creator has for us, he sent his only son to die for our sins, and when his son was about to leave, he didn't want to leave us alone so he sent someone to us. John 14:16 "And I will ask the Father, and he will give you another Helper, to be with you forever" so we are not alone we have a helper the holy spirit but the truth is that not everyone has the holy spirit because you can only have the holy spirit when you accept Jesus Christ as your Lord and saviour because you have to open the door before he enters. Revelation 3:20 "Behold, I stand at the door and knock. If anyone hears my voice and opens the door, I will come into him and eat with him, and he with me." He is currently knocking, the question is would you open the door to the one who loves you

and is more than a conquer and let him conquer depression permanently in your life, if you are ready say this prayer with me. "Lord Jesus, I confess my sins and ask for your forgiveness, I believe you are the son of God, I believe you died on the cross for my sins and resurrected, I believe that you love me and I accept you into my life as my Lord and saviour, thank you Lord Jesus for forgiving my sins and giving me eternal life"

After saying this prayer, you now have the surest person to ever have on your team with you. You can contact me or this email below to inform me of the step you just took now

Theamiesofchrist@gmail.com

Imagine having someone you can share all your secrets with not only because he already knows it but because you can trust him.

Imagine someone who created you and can recreate you, someone who can make you whole, someone who can make you who you want to be, you don't have to imagine because his name is Jesus and he is waiting for you.

WHAT YOU SHOULDN'T DO

DON'T ONE

We say a lot about things we should do but we don't mention the things we definitely shouldn't do. We can't mention everything we shouldn't do, just like we can't mention everything we should do.

DON'T DO DRUGS, DON'T DRINK ALCOHOL.

See depression is a great swimmer, trying to drown it in alcohol isn't going to help. I like how that sounds, you can quote me on that (*<_>*)

Drugs, when not prescribed by a Doctor, have been known to ruin a life, do not engage with it, don't have it around because you can be tempted, even the bible said to flee from every appearance of evil.

<u>DON'T TWO</u>

Do not commit suicide; because it cannot solve the pain, it is only going to transfer it to your loved ones, you might think you have the perfect way to escape from reality without causing your loved ones or those who love or care about you but that is only desperation trying to manifest itself from the inside of you, you are not weak for considering it, but don't ever think about it or consider it because no matter how hard it might be suicide is not an option. It is never an option

DON'T THREE

Do not drift away from those who love you, do not drift
away from those you love, because it is instinct to
want to segregate yourself, but don't there is a time to
be alone, but when depressed it is not a time to drift
away from those you love and those who love you.

MACHINE LEARNING AS A POTENTIAL SOLUTION

I gave a hint on how machine learning could potentially be a method of eradicating depression but all I gave was a hint, I did not go into details, I am not planning to go into details but I am planning to give a little more than I gave in the previous chapters.

I have a little experience in the Artificial intelligence, machine learning and deep learning world, I have worked on simple chatting bots to advance chatting bots to automated systems to create a machine learning algorithm that could identify the age and gender of humans by just looking at their ocular region in the pictures provided, the success rate was more than 80%, I would admit I did very little in the last as it was the work of a friend, Amusa Kehinde Hussain but I did learn a lot from it, I am not just trying to list my credentials to you I am only trying to give you a reason to listen to the very little thing that I have to say, obviously you are going to have to fix some of the logic.

I have learnt that machine learning can do a lot of things in today's world and we give it less credit than it deserves, we also fear it much more than we should.

THE LOGICAL CON USING ML

I have heard of a brain scanner eight times more powerful than a conventional MRI machine(You know Magnetic resonance imaging and you should know that MRI has a higher spatial resolution than electroencephalography (EEG). MRI with hyperintense lesions on FLAIR and DWI provides information related to brain activity over a longer period than a standard EEG where only controversial patterns like lateralized periodic discharges (LPDs) may be recorded). This brain scanner that I said I have heard of, well technically "read off" produces images that are four to eight times more detailed, and does so one-sixth of the time. The scanner is apparently quiet enough for a baby to sleep inside, and relies on a new brain-imaging technique called diffusion MRI, which maps long-distance white matter connections in the brain by tracking the movement of water.

Get that brain scanner, and use it in the collection of data, two groups of data will be collected. The first datum set should be The Undepressed Brain, this would contain data collected from the scans of the undepressed host, The second datum set should be The Depressed Brain.

Trying my best to be as ethical as possible, I think the host can be humans because the method of data collection is not intrusive at all the person has to give consent and a paper works should be signed to avoid legal jibber-jabbers, it is like a more advance survey and is not a type of human experimentation.

Speaking of surveys, a questionnaire can be administered to those who are going to take the brain scan to identify who will be categorized as depressed and undepressed.

Existing medical illness or/and family history can be collected as it might have a direct effect on the brain without it being depression. Depression screening instruments can be used, the purpose of all this is because the data collected must be as original as possible because the data collected is the foundation of everything.

The parameters to look out for are tracking of eye movements, pupil dilation, heartbeat, brain waves, size of inflammation, and whether or not there is inflammation in the brain(this can be recorded as a 0 and 1, 0 for no inflammation and 1 for inflammation), thickness of grey matter at a different part of the brain, amount of cortisol, the size of the hippocampus the size of the prefrontal cortex, how active the amygdala is, images of pet scans, amount of dopamine and other neurotransmitter hormones and other parameters you can think of, to advance the study the depressed brain can be classified into subsets based on the type of depression as this can help use machine learning or AI (Artificial intelligence) in determine type of depression or/and identify new types of depression.

A model should be created, you can use supervised, unsupervised, and reinforcement learning differently, CNN (Convolutional Neural Network) can be used in training any of the image models and any other image framework in machine learning. New Deep Learning algorithms can be developed and used and as many as possible existing deep/machine learning algorithms can be used, it is a very tedious process and that is why I am simply doing the talk and expecting any trained professional to do the work, but the truth is that it is worth the troubles.

This one project on conning depressing using machine learning has led to many sub-projects worthy to be called projects, we can just refer to it as one multifaceted project.

If models are created, then training should begin, then testing and be on the look for the model with the highest prediction percentage, the best model can be improved and tailored for use.

Like I said earlier there are many faulty logics which need improvement.

My View

If we at one point in our lives traded forex then we understand the meaning of leverage, don't mind me; we don't have to trade forex to understand what leverage means, in my defence how else was I going to let you know I have traded forex at one point in my life. Did I have to write a book before I got the money I may have or may have not lost, well that I am not going to say anything about.

Yeah, right leverage, I like to believe the Depression leverages on chain reactions to work best, let us get ready to put our chain reaction to con depression into action, talk about giving depression a taste of its own medicine, I am sure you have heard of "Long cons" we are about to discover that depression is, in fact, a coward.

Suggests, associated, maybes are not enough to convict someone of a crime and that is what the scientific body often uses when talking about depression it is also the reason why it is not yet in prison. But you can go rogue and be the judge, jury and executioner against depression, it is time for you the inmate to be released and make depression an inmate in the prison of your choice

Depression can be defeated, depression can be conned, communities can be built to help our fight against depression, and we can support ourselves to fight against this common enemy.

REFERENCES

- Google

- Wikipedia

- Lynette L. Craft, PhD and Frank M. Perna, Ed.D., PhD. The Benefits of Exercise for the Clinically Depressed.

- Basner M, Babisch W, Davis A, Brink M, Clark C, Janssen S, et al. Auditory and non-auditory effects of noise on health. The lancet. 2014;383(9925):1325–32. https://doi.org/10.1016/S0140-6736(13)61613-X.

- Stansfeld SA, Matheson MP. Noise pollution: non-auditory effects on health. British medical bulletin. 2003;68(1):243–57. https://doi.org/10.1093/bmb/ldg033 PMid:14757721

- Wang S, Yu Y, Feng Y, Zou F, Zhang X, Huang J, et al. Protective effect of the orientin on noise-induced cognitive impairments in mice. Behavioural brain research. 2016;296:290–300.

https://doi.org/10.1016/j.bbr.2015.09.024 PMid:26392065.

https://www.healthline.com/health/types-of-depression#seasonal-depression

https://www.medicalnewstoday.com/articles/318428#vitamin-d

https://uniquemindcare.com/7-common-types-of-depression/

https://www.beyondblue.org.au/the-facts/depression/types-of-depression

https://successtms.com/blog/types-of-depression

https://www.mayoclinic.org/diseases-conditions/persistent-depressive-disorder/symptoms-causes/syc-20350929

https://www.transformationstreatment.center/treatment/what-happens-to-the-brain-during-depression/

https://www.drugs.com/illicit/ketamine.html

https://www.yalemedicine.org/news/ketamine-depression

hopkinsmedicine.org

ucf.edupegasus/your-brain-on-music/

ABOUT THE AUTHOR

AUTHOR NAME is Modupe Ladele

Find out more at amazon.com/author/modupeladele

Facebook – facebook.com/modupeladele

Twitter – twitter.com/modupeladele

Instagram – instagram/modupeladele

Medium – Modupeladele.medium.com

Other Books By (Modupe Ladele)

I will list them when I am proud of them

CAN I ASK A FAVOUR?

If you enjoyed this book, found it useful or otherwise then I'd really appreciate it if you would post a short review on Amazon. I do read all the reviews personally so that I can continually write what people are wanting.

If you'd like to leave a review then please do

Thanks for your support!

Also please help me make this book better by contacting me with suggestions and improvements, together let's help eradicate depression. Recommend to people who you think might need it.